Juicing For Beginners
Secrets To The Health Benefits Of Juicing

30 Unique Recipes

Introduction

I want to thank you and congratulate you for downloading the book, *"Juicing For Beginners - Secrets To The Health Benefits Of Juicing, 30 Unique Recipes."*
This book has helpful information on juicing, how it benefits you, and 30 amazing juicing recipes.
If you wish to stop early aging, stay healthy, increase your immunity, and keep your digestive system healthy, you should incorporate juicing into your life. The amazing thing about juices, especially vegetable and fruit juices is that you don't task your digestive system with digesting the fiber; hence, the nutrients are absorbed almost immediately after consumption.
You can incorporate juicing in your daily lifestyle or opt to detox and go on a juice fast. Whatever, you reason for juicing, this book is the ultimate juicing guide for beginners; the book will give better insight into juicing and its amazing health benefits.
After highlighting the various juicing benefits, the book will then discuss 30 easy juice recipes you can try out at home and enjoy their amazing benefits.
Thanks again for downloading this book, I hope you enjoy it!

Table of Contents

Quick Insight Into Juicing And Its Benefits

Before we start discussing the 30 awesome juice recipes, we need to discuss juicing so you can understand its benefits. Juicing entails extracting juice from the fruit or vegetable and have the waste as the pulp, which you can use or discard. Juicing is an effective way to obtain essential nutrients (vitamins and minerals), enzymes, and phytonutrients from fruits and vegetables.

Quite often, people confuse juices and smoothies. To prepare a smoothie, you blend vegetables or fruits together or individually and mix them to get a mixture known as a 'smoothie.' To prepare smoothies, you use a blender. Juicing, on the other hand, is a little different. In juicing, you place the whole foods in a juicing machine to extract all the juice from the fruit and then discard the fiber part.

You may be wondering why juicing has gained immense popularity in the past decade, particularly since you can purchase packaged fruit juices from the store and consume fruits and veggies directly without turning them into juice form.

Well, this is because of two main reasons:

1. Commercial juices undergo a lot of processing and the large-scale manufactures fill it with preservatives, additives, and artificial flavors; this negatively changes the nutritional value of the juice. By the time the juice reaches you, it has lost much of its original nutritional value.

Many juice brands claim that their fruit juices are 100 percent fresh; this however, is not true. Juices that last longer than 3 hours or four days (when refrigerated) are full of preservatives because real fresh juices usually go bad 3 hours after extraction and a few days of refrigeration. Hence, the nutrients present in store-bought and packaged juices are no match to those in homemade juices.

2. Secondly, do you eat all the fruits and vegetables available at the supermarket? Think again. Your answer is a definable 'no'. This is one of the many reasons why juicing is a big hit: because it allows you to mix many veggies, fruits, and herbs to prepare a tasty concoction you can easily drink.

If you do not like the taste of beets or kale, you can mix it with berries and citrus fruits and enjoy the health benefits of both these veggies. As you can clearly see, juicing easily helps you enjoy the health benefits of all the different fruits, veggies, and herbs you are not a big fan of.

With that basic understanding of juicing, let us discuss its health benefits so you become motivated to try it too.

Why Juice: Benefits Of Juicing

Juicing has a number of health benefits. This chapter explores juicing different health benefits with the intent being to help you understand why this approach has become so famous and why you should adopt it.

Aids in Weight Management

Juicing is very effective in weight loss; however, contrary to popular gutter press news, this does not happen overnight. To use juicing for weight loss, you have to make juicing a habit and rely on juices for energy and nutrition.

To lose weight through juicing, you have two options. You can decide to replace some of your meals with juices or you can go for a juice fast to kick start your weight loss journey. When you go on a juice fast, you create an atmosphere of low concentration toxic wastes in the circulatory system. When this happens, your body cells slowly release different toxic wastes and since toxins are usually stored in fat, you lose fat in the processes.

You can go on a juice fast for as long as you want and are willing to. However, it is best not to prolong it to an extent that your health starts to deteriorate. It is best to start with smaller fasts of around 2 to 5 days and gradually move to longer fasts. By doing this, your body accustoms to these fasts and adjusts accordingly.

Once you commence a juice fast, you may experience the following side effects:

Dizziness: Since you are used to consuming heavy meals, when you cut back on your intake of heavy foods and drink juices instead, you may experience a lack of energy and dizziness. This is perfectly normal and usually subsides within a day or two. To manage this dizziness, slowly scale back your intake of regular meals so your body can easily adjust to juicing.

Headaches: As you start, you may experience a few headaches; again, this is perfectly normal. This happens because of the shift in your energy levels from relying more on juices than on heavy, calorie rich meals. To manage this side effect, drink plenty of water. You can also dilute your juices and turn one glass of juice into two glasses by mixing it in a glass of water. Water energizes you and helps you manage headaches.

Stick to this advice and you will find it easier to go on a juice fast.

Helps Prevent Diseases

Fresh juices are rich in phytonutrients and antioxidants. Phytonutrients and antioxidants protect your body from free radicals; free radicals are cells missing a critical molecule that are major cancer precursors. Free radicals damage the cell's DNA and start dangerous reactions in your body.

Usually, routine cellular activity generates a little amount of free radicals; however, this does not cause any health problem since your system's natural antioxidants battle these free radicals and neutralize their effect.

Problems start when you overload your body with too many free radical sources. Chemicals in packaged and processed foods, cigarette smoke, pollution, and alcohol are some of the biggest sources of free radicals.

When your free radical intake becomes too high, you need more antioxidants to effectively deal with the free radical garbage in your body. This is where juicing comes in handy. Juices are rich in lycopene, beta-carotene, quercetin, and many other antioxidants that battle the free radicals and prevent them for harming your DNA. Free radicals fight your body cells to take their molecules and in this battle, they often harm your DNA.

By neutralizing the effects of free radicals and flushing them out of your body, antioxidants ensure this does not happen and by doing so, keep you healthy and decrease your likelihood of suffering from cancer and other serious health conditions.

In addition, juices are full of enzymes that help improve your digestion process and keep you healthy. Enzymes are the compounds that break up nutrients for easy digestion. Fruits and vegetables are rich in enzymes specifically present to digest their nutrients.

For example, sucrose is an enzyme present in juicy fruits to digest sucrose and maltase present in grains and malt. Similarly, different kinds of enzymes present in different foods aid your digestive process.

When you consume fruits and vegetables in juice form, your body gets the enzymes contained in them too and this makes your digestion process easier and smoother.

Provides Energy

Vegetables and fruit juices are rich sources of electrolytes like magnesium, potassium, calcium, and sodium, electrolytes important for metabolism, stabilizing blood sugar levels, and for proper muscles and brain functioning. As these changes occur in your body, you become more energetic.

Moreover, juices are also rich in vitamins A, B and C, vitamins that boost your mental and physical energy. Further, juices are directly absorbed into your bloodstream; this means your body takes them up very fast since the body does not have to digest them before utilizing them. This means that as you drink a juice, you get an instant energy boost.

Now that you know the health benefits of juicing, let us look at how to incorporate juicing into your life.

Getting Started With Juicing

Here is how you can get started with juicing.

Step 1: Select Your Juicer

Different types of juicers are available in the market; however, we can broadly categorize most of them into two categories:

Centrifugal: These juicers are a common sight at juice bars. They use a high-speed blade to cut and crush the ingredients. The rotating action of the blade oxidizes the juice, which changes the nutritional content of the juice.

Although these juicers are economical, when compared to the other category of juicers, these often extract less juice from the produce's pulp. However, if you are on a budget, you should opt for this juicer.

Masticating & Cold Press, Double and Single Auger Juicers: These juicers crush the produce and squeeze juice out of them at a slower rate than the centrifugal ones. This leads to less oxidization, which means more nutrients extracted out of the pulp.

Hence, compared to juices extracted using a centrifugal juicer, the juices prepared using these juicers are healthier. If you can spare approximately $250 or more, buy any one of these juicers.

Once you buy a juicer, move to the next step.

Step 2: Shop for Some Grocery

Make a list of the produce you want according to the benefits you want to enjoy from juicing. If you want to use juicing to lose weight, opt for green, leafy veggies. When creating your grocery-shopping list, consider your taste palette and likes. You can use this app to create your grocery list.

As a beginner, it is best to opt for produce you enjoy eating. If you love apples, citrus fruits, and celery, buy these ingredients and prepare their juices. Add more variety once you settle into the idea of juicing and are ready to experiment.

Once you buy the produce, wash it thoroughly a night before you plan to juice or a few hours before juicing. If you are washing it a night before, rinse it well and let it dry in a basket on the kitchen counter for an hour or so. Once it completely dries, store it in the fridge.

Step 3: Start Juicing

When you are ready to juice, do the following:

1. Read your juicers' manual to get a better understanding of its operations before juicing.

2. Line your juicer's pulp basket if it has one with a plastic bag; this will make cleaning easier.

3. Cut all the produce into small pieces so they can easily fit through juicer's chute and be easier to juice. When you cut the produce, it loses nutrients; therefore, cut your produce shortly before juicing.

4. Place the cut produce in the juicer's chute and juice it. Once you juice all the produce, check its pulp. If it is damp, it means the pulp has some more juicy goodness to give. Re-juice that pulp to get more juice. When the pulp feels completely dry, it means you have extracted all the juice from it and you can now safely discard it.

Step 4: Storing Juices

Although it is best to drink juices fresh or immediately after preparation, if you are pressed for time and cannot do so, you can store your juices. Here are some tips to help you store your juice the right way.

1. Make at least two servings of a juice you want to store. Drink half of it immediately after preparing it and refrigerate the rest in an airtight container to drink later that day or the next morning.

2. Use a glass container to store juice; however, if you do not have a glass container, you can use BPA-free plastic containers.

3. Fill the container with juice until the very top to ensure oxygen does not get inside and deplete the nutrients.

4. Store the juice in the refrigerator for 24 to 48 hours. You can store it for 72 hours too, but not more than that because after 3 days, a refrigerated juice loses all its nutritional value.

5. You can freeze it too; however, compared to refrigeration, freezing is a less desirable option. To freeze a juice, do so right after preparing the juice. When you want to drink the frozen juice, thaw it in the fridge. Use the frozen juice within 7 to 10 days of freezing.

Step 5: Combining Different Ingredients

There are lots of vegetables, herbs, and even fruit you may not enjoy eating. However, if you plan to make juicing a constant in your life, and want to reap its full benefits, it is important to juice different produce.

Here are some ways to combine different ingredients and produce so you get delicious juices each time.

* Kale, spinach, and beets have strong tastes and many 'juicers' do not like juicing them. To juice these, you can combine them with cranberries, raspberries, strawberries, and citrus fruits to turn yucky into yummy.
* To add a nice flavor to different juices, add spices, extracts, and herbs like cinnamon, ginger, cilantro, basil, nutmeg, and mint.
* If you find a vegetable juice hard to swallow, add a teaspoon of honey to sweeten its bitter or strong taste.

To incorporate juices into your life, make them a permanent part of your breakfast, lunch, and snacks. Drink a glass of juice for breakfast and one or two whenever you feel hungry. This helps you stay fit and lose weight especially if you opt for a low calorie juice.

Now that you know how to start juicing, let us look at some amazing juice recipes you can start enjoying.

Yummy Fruit Juice Recipes For A Healthy Body

Let us begin with some simple fruit juice recipes for healthy body.

1. Refreshing Kiwi Juice

Serves 2
Ingredients
2 kiwifruits, cubed
1 cup of raspberries
2 cups cubed watermelon
Directions
1. Wash the fruits; place the fruits in the juicer and juice.
2. Serve, add ice, and enjoy.
Health Benefits
Kiwi's skin provides omega 3 fatty acids, which even though are essential for normal growth; your body cannot produce it. Moreover, omega-3 fatty acids provide relief from extreme depression and mania phases experienced in bipolar disorder. These essential nutrients also soothe the terrible pain caused by arthritis and lower your elevated blood pressure. Additionally, omega 3 fatty acids also improve your cardiovascular risk profile and help you fight cardiovascular disorders.

Moreover, watermelon and raspberries are full of antioxidants that keep you safe from the harmful effects of free radicals and keep your skin and hair healthy. With this juice, you will definitely enhance your health.

2. Citrus Juice

Serves 2

Ingredients

2 oranges

2 tangerines

Directions

1. Peel the fruits; place them in the juicer, and juice.

2. Serve, and enjoy your drink.

Health Benefits

This juice is the perfect combination of vitamin C and potassium, both essential nutrients that lower blood pressure, help you easily manage stress, and keep your kidneys and heart healthy.

3. Apple and Strawberry Juice

Serves 2

Ingredients

1 large red apple

250g strawberries

Ice cubes

Directions

1. Cut the apple into half and remove its core. Cut the two halves into wedges.

2. Wash the strawberries and remove their hulls.

3. Process the apples and strawberries in a juicer.

4. Pour the juice in glasses, add ice cubes, and enjoy the juicy goodness.

Health Benefits

Strawberries help cure urinary tract infections. Apples are a good source of vitamin C that helps reduce risk of cancer, diabetes, and cardiovascular conditions.

4. Fruit Cleanser

Serves 2

Ingredients

Flesh of about 1/4 seedless watermelon

½ cup cranberry juice

1 cup grape juice
Directions
1. Process the watermelon flesh in a juicer and extract its juice.
2. Pour it in a jug and add the cranberry and grape juices.
3. Mix well and pour in glasses to serve.
Health Benefits
Watermelon is rich in vitamins A, C, and B6, amino acids, and lycopene that reduce your body fat, improve cardiovascular health, strengthen your bones, and reduce inflammation in your body. Cranberry and grape juices are full of vitamin C goodness and antioxidants that strengthen your immune system by flushing out toxins from your body.

5. Beet Goodness

Serves 1
Ingredients
1 handful of raspberries
1 handful of fresh strawberries
1 beetroot
Directions
1. Cut the beet into chunks and run it run through the juicer.
2. Add the berries to the juicer and pour the mixture into a glass.
Health Benefits
Beetroot and raspberries are rich in antioxidants and as you already know, antioxidants boost your cardiac health, enhance your immune system, and reduce inflammation.

6. Apple Citrus Juice

Serves 2
Ingredients
3 peeled oranges
1 apple
½ ruby red grapefruit (peeled)
Directions

1. Thoroughly wash all the fruits.
2. Cut oranges and grapefruit into quarters and add them to the juicer.
3. At the very end, juice the apple and serve.

Health Benefits

This vitamin C and iron rich juice boosts your energy levels, and thus keeps you energetic the entire day. Moreover, with this drink, you enjoy all the various benefits of vitamin C too; benefits such as reduced inflammation and an enhanced immune system.

7. Mint Strawberry Finisher

Serves 2

Ingredients

½ large papaya
1 cup of strawberries
1 handful of fresh mint (with stalks)

Directions

1. Thoroughly wash all the ingredients.
2. Cut the papaya into cubes.
Juice the three ingredients together and drink your juice immediately.

Health Benefits

Mint keeps your digestive tract healthy and helps it digest food quickly; strawberries on the other hand have a good serving of antioxidants.

8. Orange Vanilla Juice

Serves 8

Ingredients

1 teaspoon vanilla extract
Juice of ½ lemon
250g strawberries
5 peeled oranges

Directions

1. Using your juicer, extract the juice of oranges and strawberries.
2. Add the vanilla extract and lemon juice to the orange and strawberry juice.
3. Pour into glasses and serve.

9. Coconut Pineapple Juice

Serves 1
Ingredients
2 tablespoons canned full-fat coconut milk
2 cups cubed pineapple
2 cups cubed mango
1 peeled lime with its pith and seeds removed
1 inch section galangal
1 inch ginger root
Directions
1. Pass the produce through a juicer excluding the coconut milk.
2. Pour the coconut milk in a glass and add the juice on top of it. Mix well and serve.
Try these mouthwatering fruit juices for a healthy lifestyle.
Vegetables juices are equally important as fruit juices. Let us now discuss vegetable juice recipes.

Tasteful Vegetable Juices

Vegetables rich in phytonutrients are best for juicing, and provide instant energy and pure form of nutrition. Here are some delicious and healthy vegetable juice recipes for you.

10. Green Juice

Serves 2
Ingredients
3 medium sized celery stalks
1 medium sized peeled lemon with its pith removed
2 medium sized garlic cloves
1 large carrot
4 medium sized kale leaves
1 medium sized cucumber
Frank's Red Hot or any other vinegary hot sauce you like
Directions
1. Juice the ingredients in your juicer.
2. Pour the juice into your glass and add the hot sauce.

11. Spicy Vegetable Juice

Serves 2
Ingredients
2 large sized tomatoes
¼ cup of cilantro
½ cucumber
4 stalks of celery
1 jalapeño with seeds
¼ lemon (peeled without seeds)
Directions
1. Thoroughly rinse all the vegetables.
2. Cut tomatoes into cubes and juice.
3. Add cucumber and juice.

4. Add the celery stalk, cilantro, and jalapeño to the juicer. If you want, you can juice jalapeno with the seeds.
5. Mix all the juice and serve.

Health Benefits

This spicy vegetable juice is full of beta-carotene and lycopene that reduce your risk of cardiovascular diseases and heart strokes. In addition, they boost your cellular health and enhance your liver performance.

12.   Chard and Kale Juice

Serves 4
Ingredients
1 bunch of kale
1 bunch of baby spinach
2 or 3 large leaves of Swiss chard
3 large carrots
1 large cucumber
½ lemon
2 large Granny Smith apples
Directions
1. Wash all the vegetables.
2. Slightly peel your carrots to conserve most of their nutrients. After peeling, cut them into chunks and juice them.
3. Cut the cucumber with the skin and juice it as well.
4. Add the kale, spinach, and Swiss chard leaves and juice them.
5. Remove the cores of the apples, cut them in cubes, and juice them along with half a lemon.
6. Mix all the juices and drink immediately.

Health Benefits

If you are new to juicing, this juice is appropriate because it is neither too bland nor too sweet. This juice is also full of nutrients like Vitamin C, iron, and carotene.

13.   Vegetable Juice

Serves 2
Ingredients
3 medium sized carrots
1 large or 2 small beetroots
2 stalks of fresh celery
1 inch piece of ginger
Directions
1. Wash all the produce.
2. Cut the carrots into cubes and the beetroot into half.
3. Pace all the ingredients in the juicer and juice.
4. Sere, add a few ice cubes and enjoy.
Health Benefits
Ginger is best for your digestive system and helps you combat various conditions related to digestion. It also relieves nausea, flatulence, and motion sickness.

14. Kale Juice

Serves 2
Ingredients
A dash of hot sauce
2 lemons
4 celery stalks
½ pound kale
2 pints grape or cherry tomatoes
1 tablespoon of soy sauce
Directions
1. Juice the tomatoes, kale, celery, and lemons.
2. Pour into a glass; add in hot sauce and soy sauce and mix.
3. Serve and enjoy

15. Savory Juice

Serves 1
Ingredients
1 handful of parsley
2 rainbow chard stems and leaves

2 Swiss chard stems and leaves
8 romaine lettuce leaves
2 celery stalks
4 tomatoes
A pinch of pepper and salt
Dash of Tabasco

Directions

1. Wash the produce and juice.
2. Pour the juice into a glass and top it with hot sauce, pepper, and salt.

So far, we have discussed many fruit and vegetable juices. Now need to look at a few recipes of mixed vegetable, fruit, and herb juices. If you love the combination of fruits and vegetables, you will enjoy these recipes. Move to the next chapter to enjoy those recipes.

Mixed Fruit And Vegetable Juices

Fruit, vegetables, and spices together perform miracles for you overall health. Moreover, their flavors blend well and result in delicious juices. Here are some amazing mix fruit, veggies, herbs and spices juicing recipes for you.

16. Apple Beet Juice

Serves 1
Ingredients
1 apple
3 medium sized carrots
1/2 beetroot
Directions
1. Wash all the ingredients.
2. Cut the apples, carrots, and beetroots into chunks.
3. Remove the cores of the apple before juicing.
4. Juice, serve, add ice, and enjoy.
Health Benefits
The Beetroot in this juice provides fiber, protein, iron, and antioxidants. The carrots give you calcium, while apples provide all the essential vitamins and iron.

17. Tropical Juice

Serves 1
Ingredients
1 apple
2 pineapple spears
½ lemon (without peel)
2 carrots
Directions
1. Thoroughly wash your apples, lemon, and carrots.
2. Cut the carrots into chunks.
3. Cut the apples into halves and remove their cores.

4. Juice all the ingredients, serve, and enjoy.
Health Benefits
Pineapple gives an extra fresh flavor to the drink along with calcium and antioxidants. This juice is also ideal for children since it is sweet.

18.   Green Apple Juice

Serves 1
Ingredients
1 handful of kale
1 spear of pineapple
2 Granny smith apples
¼ lemon
Directions
1. Wash the kale, lemon, and apples.
2. Peel the lemon and remove the seeds.
3. Cut the apple into cubes and remove its core.
4. Juice all the ingredients, serve, add ice, and enjoy.
Health Benefits
Green leafy vegetables like kale provide good fiber and calcium that improves your heart's health.

19.   Apple and Broccoli Juice

Serves 2
Ingredients
1 lemon with its rind and skin removed
1 cup broccoli florets
4 large unpeeled, chopped, and cored Granny smith apples
Directions
1. Process all the ingredients in a juicer.
2. Serve the juice, add ice if you want and enjoy.
Health Benefits

Broccoli is one of the best foods in the world. It is rich in pantothenic acid, vitamins A, B-complex and E, copper, potassium, manganese, and phosphorus, which helps you fight cancer, improve bone health, and prevent early aging. Lemon juice is full of vitamin C that removes toxins from the body.

20. Minty Apple Juice

Serves 8
Ingredients
1 peeled lime
2 cups of mint leaves
100g baby spinach leaves
4 celery stalks
5 green apples
Directions
1. Process all the ingredients in a juicer.
2. Serve the juice and enjoy.
Health Benefits
Spinach is full of vitamins A, K, C, and E, thiamin, folate, iron, magnesium, manganese, phosphorus, and several other nutrients that make it effective at fighting cancer, lowering high blood pressure, and enhancing the health of your skin and hair.

21. Apple Celery Juice

Serves 4
Ingredients
5cm peeled and sliced piece of fresh ginger
6 Granny smith apples
6 trimmed celery stalks
Directions
1. Cut the apples into wedges and remove their cores.
2. Juice the ingredients, serve, add ice if you want and enjoy.
Health Benefits

Ginger has 'gingerol,' the compound that helps it fight diseases and heals injuries fast.

22. Cucumber Strawberry Juice

Serves 2
Ingredients
6 fresh strawberries (hulled)
1 large red apple
1 peeled cucumber
2 peeled medium carrots
Directions
1. Cut the cucumber into chunks and the apple into wedges.
2. First process the strawberries in the juicer followed by cucumber, apple, and then carrots.
3. Pour the juice into glasses and serve.

23. Cool Cucumber Juice

Serves 1
Ingredients
3 stalks of fresh celery
½ cucumber
1 apple
Directions
1. Wash all the ingredients.
2. Juice the celery first followed by the cucumber.
3. Cut the apples into halves and remove the core before juicing.
4. Stir the juice to mix, pour in a glass, add ice and enjoy.
Health Benefits
Cucumber and apples provide a mixture of essential nutrients and phytonutrients.

24. Peachy Green Juice

Serves 1
Ingredients

1 bunch of kale or spinach

3 peaches

Directions

1. Cut the peaches into halves and remove the pits. Run them through the juicer.

2. Add the kale and juice.

3. Stir the juice, pour in a glass and enjoy.

Health Benefits

This juice is a great source of vitamin A and E.

25. Tropical Green Juice

Serves 2

Ingredients

1 large mango, peeled and pitted

8 ounces fresh spinach

1/3 medium pineapple, peeled

1-2 limes, peeled

Directions

1. Juice all the ingredients in your juice.

2. Serve and enjoy.

Health Benefits

Mango lowers blood cholesterol, improves the digestion process, and helps fight heat stroke.

26. Sweet Potato Juice

Serves 2

Ingredients

1-2 large oranges

1 lime

1 large carrot

1 medium sized sweet potato, peeled

Directions

1. Wash the ingredients.

2. Juice the sweet potato, then the lime, carrot and finally the oranges.

3. Serve and enjoy.
Health Benefits
Sweet potatoes are high in vitamin B-complex and vitamin A, riboflavin, niacin, and thiamin. They help control your blood sugar, have anti-inflammatory properties, and improve the digestion process.

27. Basil Pear Juice

Serves 2
Ingredients
4 large celery stalks
2 peeled lemons with pith removed
2 packed cups of basil stems and leaves
4 pears
Directions
1. Process the ingredients in your juicer.
2. Mix the juice, serve, and enjoy.

28. Cucumber and Watermelon Juice

Serves 2
Ingredients
1-2 limes
15 mint leaves
1 large cucumber
6 cups of watermelon flesh
1 tablespoon sugar (optional)
Directions
1. Pass the produce through a juicer to extract the juice. You can add sugar to the juice if you want.
2. Pour into glasses and serve.

29. Tangy Pear Juice

Serves 1
Ingredients
2 ripe Anjou pears (quartered and cored)

¼ ounce of peeled ginger root

12 kumquats

Directions

1. Start by extracting the juice of the ginger followed by kumquats and pears.

2. Mix well and pour into a glass to serve.

Health Benefits

Kumquats improve your skin and digestive health, help you fight off diabetes, and strengthen your immune system.

30.   Power Potion

Serves 2

Ingredients

1 quartered and cored large apple

2 peeled clementines

1 inch piece ginger root

2 medium sized carrots

2 medium sized beets

Directions

1. Juice the ingredients.

2. Pour the juice into two glasses and serve immediately.

Try these delicious juice recipes to detoxify your body.

Conclusion

Thank you again for downloading this book!
This book has provided you with 30 amazing juice recipes that
are easy to juice. This book has also given you sufficient and
helpful knowledge on how to juice, and how juicing helps you
live a healthier life.
The ball is now in your court. Start incorporating juicing into
your life and you will immediately start living a healthier,
happier, and amazing life.

Finally, if you enjoyed this book, would you be kind enough
to leave a review for this book on Amazon?

Click here to leave a review for this book on Amazon!
Thank you and good luck!

Check Out My Other Books

Below you'll find some of my other popular books that are popular on Amazon and Kindle as well. Simply click on the links below to check them out. Alternatively, you can visit my author page on Amazon to see other work done by me.

Meditation: Meditation For Beginners How To Relieve Stress, Anxiety And Depression, Find Inner Peace And Happiness

If the links do not work, for whatever reason, you can simply search for these titles on the Amazon website to find them.